BLOW JOB
COUPONS

I0429596

By Kandy L Long

Copyright © 2016 Kandy L Long

All rights reserved.

ISBN:10: 1530596998
ISBN-13: 978-1530596997

Tear Out The Coupons To Redeem

This Coupons is

For

Blowjob In The Morning

Back Side Of Coupon

This Coupons is

For

Blowjob In The Middle of the night

Back Side
Of
Coupon

This Coupons is

For

Blowjob In The afternoon

Back
Side Of
Coupon

This Coupons is

For

Blowjob In The Evening

Back Side
Of Coupon

This Coupons is

For

Blowjob while eating lunch

Back Side Of Coupon

This Coupons is

For

Blowjob while eating dinner

Back Side Of Coupon

This Coupons is

For

Blowjob while watching Television

BACKSIDE OF
COUPON

This Coupons is

For

Blowjob while
playing video
games

Back
Side Of
Coupon

This Coupons is

For

Blowjob while
taking a shower

Back Side
Of
Coupon

This Coupons is

For

Blowjob while in the car

Back Side Of Coupon

This Coupons is

For

Blowjob while
taking a nap

Back
Side
Of
Coupon

This Coupons is

For

Blowjob anytime I want anywhere

Back Side Of Of Coupon

www.ingramcontent.com/pod-product-compliance
Lightning Source LLC
Chambersburg PA
CBHW072014280526
45788CB00005B/2035

* 9 7 8 1 5 3 0 5 9 6 9 9 7 *